ULCERATIVE COLITIS DIET COOK BOOK

A Complete Ulcerative Colitis Diet: How to Reduce Gut Inflammation and Improve Total Gut Health

LARRY HERMAN

Table of Contents

Introduction

The rectum and colon are the most common sites of damage in ulcerative colitis, a chronic inflammatory bowel disease. Diet has a significant role in symptom management and general health promotion for those with ulcerative colitis. Dietary recommendations may aid in symptom management and quality of life enhancement for individuals suffering from ulcerative colitis; however, there is no silver bullet because the effects of individual foods might differ from person to person.

• **The Low-Residue Diet:** This eating plan is centered around limiting high-fiber foods since they can aggravate bowel issues. It consists of refined grains, delicate lean meats, and vegetables that are prepared to perfection.

• Stay Away from Foods That Set You off It is Critical to Recognize Which Foods Set You Off and To Avoid Them. Dairy products, spicy food, coffee, alcohol, and meals high in fiber are common triggers.

• **Eat Small, Regular Meals:** It is easier for the digestive system to eat smaller meals throughout the day instead of a few big ones, which can help with symptom management.

• **Hydration:** People suffering with ulcerative colitis should make sure to drink plenty of water because the inflammation and diarrhea can cause them to become dehydrated. One way to keep fluid levels stable is to drink lots of water.

- **Foods Rich in Omega-3 Fatty Acids:** Oily fish (salmon, mackerel), flaxseeds, and walnuts are good sources of omega-3 fatty acids, which may help with symptom management because of their anti-inflammatory characteristics.

- **Probiotics:** Some yoghurts and pills contain probiotics, which can help maintain a balanced population of gut bacteria and may be useful for symptom control.

7. Calcium and vitamin D: People with ulcerative colitis could have trouble absorbing minerals, so it's vital to make sure they get enough calcium and vitamin D to keep their bones healthy. Particularly in cases of lactose intolerance, supplements could be required.

Individuals with ulcerative colitis must collaborate closely with their healthcare team, which should include a certified dietitian, to create a tailored eating plan that addresses their unique requirements. be little changes to your diet at first, and talk to your doctor before making any major changes to be sure they fit in with your treatment plan.

CHAPTER ONE
What is Ulcerative Colitis?

Ulcerative colitis is a persistent inflammatory condition of the colon and rectum, categorized as an inflammatory bowel disease (IBD). It is distinguished by inflammation and the formation of ulcers in the inner lining of the colon, resulting in various symptoms and possible problems. The precise etiology of ulcerative colitis remains uncertain, while it is thought to result from a complex interplay of genetic, environmental, and immunological factors.

Notable characteristics of ulcerative colitis include:

• Ulcerative colitis is characterized by inflammation that initially occurs in the rectum and can then spread constantly throughout the colon. The intensity of inflammation can vary, and it may affect various layers of the intestinal wall.

• **Ulcers:** Inflammation in the colon can lead to the formation of open sores or ulcers, which can worsen the symptoms and complications of the illness.

• **Symptoms:** Typical manifestations of ulcerative colitis are abdominal discomfort, diarrhea (often accompanied by blood or pus), rectal bleeding, an urgent need to defecate, and a continuous sensation of needing to evacuate the bowels. Additionally, fatigue, weight loss, and diminished appetite may occur.

• Ulcerative colitis typically follows a relapsing-remitting pattern, where patients go through cycles of active symptoms (flare-ups) and periods of diminished or no symptoms (remission).

• **Complications:** Severe instances of ulcerative colitis can result in complications such as inflammation extending beyond the colon, which can impact other areas of the body, as well as an elevated susceptibility to colon cancer.

• The chronic nature and unpredictable course of ulcerative colitis can have a substantial influence on an individual's quality of life. Effective symptom management typically necessitates medical intervention, modifications to one's lifestyle, and occasionally surgical intervention.

• The diagnosis of ulcerative colitis is made by utilizing a comprehensive approach that includes reviewing the patient's medical history, conducting a physical examination, performing blood tests, utilizing imaging investigations, and conducting endoscopic procedures, such as colonoscopy, to inspect the interior of the colon and collect tissue samples for study.

Possible treatment modalities for ulcerative colitis may encompass pharmacological interventions aimed at regulating inflammation, alleviating symptoms, and modulating the immune response. In certain instances, surgical intervention, such as colon removal, may be advised if medicinal treatment is inadequate or if complications arise. Collaboration between persons suffering from ulcerative colitis and healthcare experts is crucial in order to create a thorough and personalized treatment strategy.

Causes and Triggers

The exact cause of ulcerative colitis is not well understood, and it likely involves a combination of genetic, environmental, and immunological factors. While researchers continue to investigate the precise triggers, several factors may contribute to the development and exacerbation of ulcerative colitis:

1. **Genetic Factors:** There is a genetic component to ulcerative colitis, as it tends to run in families. Individuals with a family history of inflammatory

bowel disease (IBD) are at a higher risk of developing ulcerative colitis. However, the majority of people with the condition do not have a family history.

2. **Immune System Dysfunction:** Ulcerative colitis is considered an autoimmune disease, where the immune system mistakenly attacks the cells of the digestive tract. The inflammation seen in the colon and rectum is a result of an abnormal immune response.

3. **Environmental Factors:** Environmental factors may play a role in triggering ulcerative colitis in genetically

predisposed individuals. Factors such as infections, exposure to certain microbes or viruses, and changes in the gut microbiota have been investigated as potential environmental triggers.

4. **Smoking:** Smoking has been identified as a factor that may influence the development and course of ulcerative colitis. While it appears to be a protective factor against developing ulcerative colitis, it is associated with a more severe disease course once the condition is established.

5. **Stress and Lifestyle:** While stress does not cause ulcerative

colitis, it can exacerbate symptoms and contribute to flare-ups. Adopting a healthy lifestyle, managing stress, and getting adequate sleep can help in managing the condition.

6. **Dietary Factors:** Certain foods may act as triggers for some individuals with ulcerative colitis. Common triggers include high-fiber foods, dairy products, spicy foods, and caffeine. However, the impact of specific foods can vary among individuals, and it's important for each person to identify their own dietary triggers through trial and observation.

7. **Infections:** Gastrointestinal infections may be linked to the onset of ulcerative colitis in some cases. The body's immune response to an infection may trigger an abnormal inflammatory response in the colon.

It's important to note that while these factors may contribute to the development or exacerbation of ulcerative colitis, the disease is complex and varies widely among individuals. Each person's experience with ulcerative colitis is unique, and the interplay of genetic and environmental factors can differ from one case to another. Research is ongoing to better understand the specific mechanisms and triggers of ulcerative colitis, which may lead to more targeted and effective treatments in the future.

CHAPTER TWO
Diagnosis and Treatment Options

Diagnosing and treating ulcerative colitis typically involves a combination of clinical evaluation, diagnostic procedures, and a comprehensive treatment plan. Here's an overview of the diagnosis and treatment options for ulcerative colitis:

Diagnosis:

1. **Medical History and Physical Examination:**
   - A detailed medical history is taken to understand symptoms, family history, and overall health.

- A physical examination helps assess abdominal tenderness, signs of malnutrition, and other relevant symptoms.

2. **Blood Tests:**

   - Blood tests may be conducted to check for signs of inflammation, anemia, and nutritional deficiencies.

3. **Stool Sample Analysis:**

   - Analyzing a stool sample can help rule out infections and provide information about inflammation in the digestive tract.

4. **Endoscopic Procedures:**

- o **Colonoscopy:** A thin, flexible tube with a camera (colonoscope) is used to visualize the entire colon and rectum. Tissue samples (biopsies) may be taken for further analysis.

- o **Flexible Sigmoidoscopy:** Similar to a colonoscopy but focuses on the lower part of the colon and rectum.

5. **Imaging Studies:**

- o X-rays, CT scans, or MRI may be used to visualize the digestive tract and assess the extent and severity of inflammation.

Treatment:

1. **Medications:**
   - **Anti-Inflammatory Drugs:** Aminosalicylates, such as mesalamine, are often prescribed to reduce inflammation and maintain remission.
   - **Corticosteroids:** Short-term use of steroids like prednisone may be recommended during flare-ups to control severe inflammation.
   - **Immunomodulators:** Medications like azathioprine or methotrexate may be

used to modify the immune system response.

- **Biologics:** Targeted therapies, such as anti-TNF agents (infliximab, adalimumab), may be prescribed for moderate to severe cases.

2. **Symptom Management:**

- Anti-diarrheal medications may be recommended to manage diarrhea.

- Pain relievers and antispasmodic medications can help alleviate abdominal pain and cramping.

3. **Dietary Changes:**
   - A low-residue diet or elimination of specific trigger foods may help manage symptoms.
   - Nutritional supplements may be recommended to address deficiencies.

4. **Lifestyle Modifications:**
   - Stress management and regular exercise can contribute to overall well-being.
   - Smoking cessation is advised, as smoking can worsen the condition.

5. **Surgery:**
   - In cases of severe complications or when

medical therapy is inadequate, surgical options may include removing the entire colon (colectomy) with or without creating an ileostomy.

6. **Monitoring and Follow-up:**

   o Regular monitoring through clinical evaluations, blood tests, and imaging helps assess disease activity and adjust treatment as needed.

   o Long-term management aims at achieving and maintaining remission to improve the individual's quality of life.

The treatment plan for ulcerative colitis is highly individualized, taking into account the severity of symptoms, disease location, and response to medications. Close collaboration between individuals with ulcerative colitis and their healthcare team, including gastroenterologists and dietitians, is crucial for effective management and optimizing long-term outcomes.

Symptoms and Complications

Ulcerative colitis presents with a variety of symptoms, ranging from mild to severe. The symptoms can fluctuate over time, with periods of active disease (flare-ups) and periods of remission. Common symptoms of ulcerative colitis include:

1. **Abdominal Pain:** Cramping and discomfort in the abdominal area, often in the lower left side.

2. **Diarrhea:** Frequent, urgent bowel movements with loose or watery stools. Blood or pus may be present in the stool.

3. **Rectal Bleeding:** Blood in the stool or on toilet paper is a

common symptom, often due to inflammation and ulcers in the rectum.

4. **Urgency to Have Bowel Movements:** A sudden and strong need to have a bowel movement, which can be difficult to control.

5. **Fatigue:** Chronic inflammation and the body's response to it can lead to fatigue and a general feeling of weakness.

6. **Weight Loss:** Loss of appetite and nutrient malabsorption can result in weight loss.

7. **Fever:** In some cases, fever may occur during flare-ups, indicating systemic inflammation.

8. **Joint Pain:** Joint pain and swelling, especially in the larger joints, can be associated with ulcerative colitis.

Complications:

1. **Severe Bleeding:** Chronic inflammation and ulcers can lead to significant bleeding, resulting in anemia and fatigue.

2. **Toxic Megacolon:** In rare cases, the colon can become severely distended, leading to a condition called toxic megacolon. This is a medical emergency and requires immediate intervention.

3. **Perforation:** Inflammation can weaken the walls of the colon,

increasing the risk of perforation, which can be a life-threatening complication.

4. **Colon Strictures:** Scar tissue formation from chronic inflammation may lead to narrowing of the colon, causing bowel obstruction.

5. **Increased Cancer Risk:** Individuals with long-standing ulcerative colitis have a slightly higher risk of developing colorectal cancer. Regular surveillance and monitoring are essential to detect any signs of dysplasia (precancerous changes) early.

6. **Extraintestinal Manifestations:** Ulcerative

colitis can affect other parts of the body, leading to complications such as joint problems, skin rashes, and eye inflammation.

7. **Osteoporosis:** Long-term use of corticosteroids and malabsorption of nutrients can contribute to decreased bone density.

It's important for individuals experiencing symptoms of ulcerative colitis to seek medical attention promptly. Timely diagnosis and appropriate treatment can help manage symptoms, reduce inflammation, and prevent or address complications. Healthcare professionals, including gastroenterologists, play a crucial role in evaluating symptoms, conducting diagnostic tests, and developing a comprehensive treatment plan tailored to the individual's specific needs and disease severity. Regular monitoring and follow-up are essential for ongoing management and maintaining a good quality of life.

CHAPTER THREE
How Diet Affects Ulcerative Colitis

Diet plays a significant role in the management of ulcerative colitis, as certain foods can either exacerbate symptoms or contribute to overall gut health. While the impact of specific foods can vary among individuals, here are some general considerations regarding how diet affects ulcerative colitis:

Foods to Consider:

• **Low-Residue Diet:** A low-residue diet reduces the intake of high-fiber foods, which can be irritating to the inflamed colon. This includes avoiding raw fruits and vegetables, whole grains, and nuts.

• **Lean Proteins:** Incorporating lean protein sources, such as poultry, fish, and well-cooked eggs, can provide essential nutrients without excessive irritation to the digestive tract.

• **Cooked Vegetables:** Cooked vegetables are generally better tolerated than raw ones. Steaming or boiling vegetables can make them easier to digest.

• **White Rice and Refined Grains:** White rice and refined grains are part of a low-residue diet and are often easier on the digestive system than whole grains.

• **Dairy Alternatives:** Some individuals with ulcerative colitis may be lactose intolerant or sensitive to dairy products. Consider lactose-free or dairy alternatives.

• **Hydration:** Staying well-hydrated is crucial, especially during flare-ups and episodes of diarrhea. Water helps maintain fluid balance and prevent dehydration.

• **Probiotics:** Probiotics, found in certain yogurts or supplements, may help promote a healthy balance of gut bacteria, potentially contributing to improved symptoms.

Foods to Limit or Avoid:

• **High-Fiber Foods:** High-fiber foods, such as whole grains, raw fruits, and vegetables, can be challenging to digest and may worsen symptoms during flare-ups.

• **Spicy Foods:** Spicy foods can be irritating to the digestive tract and may trigger symptoms like abdominal pain and diarrhea.

• **Caffeine and Alcohol:** Both caffeine and alcohol can stimulate the digestive system and may exacerbate symptoms. Limiting or avoiding these substances may be beneficial.

• **Dairy Products:** Some individuals with ulcerative colitis are lactose intolerant or sensitive to dairy.

Monitoring dairy intake and choosing lactose-free options can help.

• **Artificial Sweeteners:** Some artificial sweeteners, like sorbitol and mannitol, may cause gastrointestinal symptoms and should be limited.

• **High-Fat Foods:** High-fat foods may contribute to diarrhea and should be consumed in moderation.

Individualized Approach:

It's important to note that the impact of specific foods can vary widely among individuals with ulcerative colitis. What works for one person may not work for another. Keeping a food diary and working with a healthcare professional or registered dietitian can help identify personal triggers and develop an individualized diet plan.

During flare-ups, a more restrictive diet may be necessary to manage symptoms, while periods of remission may allow for a more varied and balanced diet. Overall, maintaining good nutrition, avoiding known triggers, and staying hydrated are essential components of dietary management for individuals with ulcerative colitis. Always consult with healthcare professionals before making significant dietary changes.

Benefits of a Well-Planned Diet

A well-planned diet can offer numerous benefits for individuals with ulcerative colitis, helping to manage symptoms, promote healing, and improve overall quality of life. Here are some key benefits:

• **Reduced Symptoms:** A diet tailored to the individual's needs can help reduce symptoms such as abdominal pain, diarrhea, and rectal bleeding. Avoiding trigger foods and focusing on easily digestible, low-residue options can minimize gastrointestinal discomfort.

• **Improved Nutritional Status:** Ulcerative colitis can lead to malabsorption of nutrients and deficiencies in vitamins and minerals. A well-balanced diet can help ensure adequate intake of essential nutrients, promoting overall health and supporting the body's healing process.

- **Maintenance of Healthy Weight:** Flare-ups of ulcerative colitis can lead to weight loss due to decreased appetite and nutrient malabsorption. A well-planned diet can help individuals maintain a healthy weight by providing nourishing, calorie-dense foods.

- **Optimized Gut Health:** Certain dietary components, such as probiotics and prebiotics found in fermented foods, fruits, and vegetables, can support a healthy balance of gut bacteria. This may help reduce inflammation and promote healing in the digestive tract.

• **Reduced Risk of Complications:** By minimizing inflammation and supporting gut health, a well-planned diet may help reduce the risk of complications associated with ulcerative colitis, such as toxic megacolon, perforation, and colorectal cancer.

• **Enhanced Immune Function:** Nutrient-rich foods and a balanced diet can support the body's immune function, helping to fight off infections and reduce the frequency and severity of flare-ups.

• **Improved Quality of Life:** Managing ulcerative colitis through diet can lead to improved overall quality of life by reducing symptoms, increasing energy levels, and promoting a sense of well-being and control over the condition.

• **Complementary to Medical Treatment:** A well-planned diet should complement medical treatment for ulcerative colitis, working synergistically with medications to manage symptoms and promote long-term remission.

• **Personalized Approach:** Every individual with ulcerative colitis may respond differently to dietary interventions. A personalized diet plan, developed in collaboration with a healthcare professional or registered dietitian, can take into account individual preferences, triggers, and nutritional needs.

Overall, a well-planned diet is a crucial component of comprehensive management for individuals with ulcerative colitis. By optimizing nutrition, supporting gut health, and minimizing symptom triggers, a tailored diet can play a significant role in improving outcomes and enhancing quality of life.

Building a Foundation: Principles of a Ulcerative Colitis-Friendly Diet

Building a foundation for an ulcerative colitis-friendly diet involves incorporating principles that aim to manage symptoms, promote gut health, and provide adequate nutrition. It's important to note that individual responses to specific foods can vary, so working with a healthcare professional or registered dietitian is essential to tailor dietary recommendations. Here are some general principles:

1. **Low-Residue Diet:**

- Focus on easily digestible foods to reduce the workload on the digestive system.
- Limit high-fiber foods, such as whole grains, raw fruits, and vegetables, during flare-ups.

2. **Small, Frequent Meals:**

- Eat smaller, more frequent meals throughout the day to minimize the impact on the digestive tract.

3. **Hydration:**

- Stay well-hydrated to prevent dehydration, especially during episodes of diarrhea.

4. Lean Proteins:

- Include lean protein sources such as poultry, fish, eggs, and tofu.

5. Cooked Vegetables:

- Choose cooked vegetables over raw ones, as they are generally gentler on the digestive system.

6. Limit Dairy:

- Monitor dairy intake, as some individuals with ulcerative colitis may be lactose intolerant. Consider lactose-free or dairy alternatives.

7. **Probiotics:**

- Incorporate probiotic-rich foods (e.g., yogurt with live cultures) or consider probiotic supplements to support a healthy balance of gut bacteria.

8. **Omega-3 Fatty Acids:**

- Include sources of omega-3 fatty acids, such as fatty fish (salmon, mackerel), flaxseeds, and walnuts, which may have anti-inflammatory effects.

9. **Limit Caffeine and Alcohol:**

- Reduce or avoid caffeine and alcohol, as they can stimulate the digestive system and exacerbate symptoms.

10. **Individualized Approach:**

- Keep a food diary to identify personal triggers and tailor the diet accordingly.
- Pay attention to specific foods that worsen symptoms during flare-ups.

11. **Nutritional Supplements:**

- Consider nutritional supplements, such as iron, calcium, and vitamin D, to address potential deficiencies.

12. **Avoid Trigger Foods:**

- Identify and avoid specific trigger foods that exacerbate symptoms. Common triggers may include spicy foods, high-fat foods, and certain artificial sweeteners.

13. **Consultation with Healthcare Professionals:**

- Collaborate with healthcare professionals, including gastroenterologists and dietitians, for personalized guidance and ongoing support.

14. **Long-Term Management:**

- Establish a long-term dietary plan that considers both symptom management during flare-ups and maintenance of remission.

15. **Balanced Nutrition:**

- Aim for a well-balanced diet that includes a variety of nutrient-dense foods to support overall health.

Building a foundation for an ulcerative colitis-friendly diet involves a combination of dietary modifications, lifestyle adjustments, and ongoing monitoring. Regular communication with healthcare professionals is crucial to ensure that the diet aligns with the individual's specific needs, and adjustments can be made based on symptom changes and overall health.

CHAPTER FOUR
Foods to Include in an Ulcerative Colitis Diet

An ulcerative colitis diet should focus on easily digestible, nutrient-dense foods that help manage symptoms and promote overall health. While individual responses to specific foods vary, here are some generally well-tolerated foods that may be included in an ulcerative colitis-friendly diet:

1. **Low-Fiber Grains:**

- White rice
- White bread
- Plain crackers
- Refined pasta

2. **Lean Proteins:**

- Skinless poultry (chicken, turkey)
- Fish (salmon, cod, trout)
- Eggs
- Tofu

3. **Cooked Vegetables:**

- Cooked carrots
- Mashed potatoes (without skins)
- Zucchini
- Butternut squash

4. **Fruits (in moderation):**

- Bananas
- Applesauce

- Peeled and cooked fruits (e.g., stewed apples)

5. Dairy Alternatives:

- Lactose-free milk
- Almond milk
- Coconut milk (if tolerated)

6. Probiotic-rich Foods:

- Yogurt with live cultures
- Kefir

7. Omega-3 Fatty Acids:

- Fatty fish (salmon, mackerel)
- Flaxseeds
- Walnuts

8. **Nut Butters:**

- Smooth nut butters (without added seeds or fibers)

9. **Cooking Oils:**

- Olive oil
- Canola oil

10. **Well-cooked and Peeled Vegetables:**

- Spinach (well-cooked)
- Green beans
- Peas

11. **Low-Fiber Fruits:**

- Cantaloupe
- Honeydew melon
- Avocado (in moderation)

12. **Refined Sugars:**

- Refined sugar in moderation
- Jellies and jams without seeds

13. **Soups and Broths:**

- Clear broths
- Blended soups without chunks or fibers

14. **Hydration:**

- Water
- Herbal teas (non-caffeinated)

15. **Nutritional Supplements:**

- Iron supplements (if needed for anemia)

- Calcium and vitamin D supplements (if advised by a healthcare professional)

16. Peanut Butter (in moderation):

- Smooth peanut butter, if tolerated

17. Well-cooked Eggs:

- Scrambled or boiled eggs

18. Grilled or Baked Chicken:

- Skinless, boneless chicken breasts

19. Quinoa (in moderation):

- Cooked quinoa

20. **Applesauce (unsweetened):**

- Unsweetened applesauce

It's important to note that individual responses to foods can vary, and it may be beneficial to keep a food diary to track how specific items affect symptoms. Additionally, dietary recommendations should be discussed with a healthcare professional or registered dietitian who can provide personalized guidance based on the individual's health status and specific needs. Adjustments to the diet may be necessary during flare-ups, and gradual reintroduction of foods during remission can be explored under guidance.

Foods to Avoid or Limit with Ulcerative Colitis

Individuals with ulcerative colitis often find relief from symptoms by avoiding or limiting certain foods that can exacerbate inflammation or irritate the digestive tract. While triggers can vary among individuals, here are some common foods to consider avoiding or limiting in an ulcerative colitis diet:

1. High-Fiber Foods:

- Whole grains (e.g., whole wheat bread, oats)
- Bran
- Seeds (e.g., flaxseeds, chia seeds)

- Nuts and nut butters with seeds

2. Raw Fruits and Vegetables:

- Raw fruits with skins or seeds (e.g., apples, berries)
- Raw vegetables (e.g., broccoli, cabbage)
- Tough or fibrous vegetables (e.g., celery, kale)

3. Spicy Foods:

- Spicy sauces and condiments (e.g., hot sauce, chili peppers)
- Spicy snacks (e.g., hot chips, salsa)

4. Dairy Products:

- Milk

- Cheese

- Ice cream

- Yogurt with active cultures (if lactose intolerant)

5. High-Fat Foods:

- Fried foods

- Fatty cuts of meat

- Creamy sauces and gravies

6. Caffeine and Alcohol:

- Coffee

- Tea (especially caffeinated)

- Carbonated drinks (e.g., soda)

- Alcohol (especially beer and wine)

7. Sugar Alcohols and Artificial Sweeteners:

- Sorbitol
- Mannitol
- Xylitol
- Sucralose

8. Tough Meats:

- Tough cuts of meat (e.g., steak)
- Processed meats (e.g., sausages, deli meats)

9. High-Fiber Snacks:

- Popcorn
- Granola bars
- Trail mix

10. Certain Spices and Condiments:

- Mustard
- Horseradish
- Vinegar-based dressings and sauces

11. High-Lactose Foods:

- Milk-based desserts (e.g., pudding, custard)
- Cream-based soups and sauces

12. Raw or Undercooked Eggs:

- Raw or undercooked eggs (e.g., in Caesar salad dressing, raw cookie dough)

13. Whole Beans and Legumes:

- Whole beans (e.g., kidney beans, chickpeas)
- Lentils

14. High-Fiber Breakfast Cereals:

- Whole-grain cereals
- Bran cereals

15. Excessive Fiber Supplements:

- Psyllium husk
- Methylcellulose
- Fiber gummies or capsules

16. Processed Foods:

- Processed snacks (e.g., chips, crackers)

- Convenience foods (e.g., frozen meals)

17. Tough Skins and Seeds:

- Tough skins of fruits (e.g., apple skins)
- Seeds in fruits and vegetables (e.g., berries, tomatoes)

18. Gassy Vegetables:

- Gas-producing vegetables (e.g., onions, cabbage, cauliflower)

19. Excessive Sugars:

- High-sugar foods and beverages
- Candy and sweets

20. Artificial Additives and Preservatives:

- Foods with artificial colors, flavors, and preservatives
- Packaged snacks and processed foods

Individual responses to these foods can vary, so it's important for individuals with ulcerative colitis to keep a food diary and pay attention to how specific foods affect their symptoms. Working with a healthcare professional or registered dietitian can provide personalized guidance and support in managing diet-related triggers and symptoms.

CHAPTER FIVE
Meal Planning and Preparation Tips

Meal planning and preparation can play a significant role in managing ulcerative colitis by ensuring that individuals have access to nourishing, well-tolerated foods. Here are some meal planning and preparation tips for individuals with ulcerative colitis:

1. **Plan Balanced Meals:** Aim to include a balance of carbohydrates, proteins, and fats in each meal to provide essential nutrients and support overall health.

2. Choose Low-Fiber Options: Opt for easily digestible, low-fiber foods such as white rice, cooked vegetables, and lean proteins to minimize digestive discomfort.

3. **Portion Control:** Eat smaller, more frequent meals throughout the day to avoid overwhelming the digestive system and minimize symptoms.

4. **Keep a Food Diary:** Keep track of foods that trigger symptoms or worsen flare-ups to identify patterns and make informed dietary choices.

5. **Meal Prep in Advance:** Prepare meals and snacks in advance to have nutritious options readily available,

especially during busy times or when experiencing fatigue.

6. **Focus on Easy-to-Digest Foods:** Choose foods that are easy to chew, swallow, and digest, such as well-cooked grains, tender meats, and soft fruits.

7. **Cook Foods Thoroughly:** Cook foods thoroughly to break down fibers and make them easier to digest, especially vegetables and meats.

8. **Experiment with Cooking Methods:** Explore different cooking methods such as steaming, boiling, baking, and grilling to find what works best for you.

9. Include Gut-Friendly Foods: Incorporate gut-friendly foods such as yogurt with live cultures, kefir, and fermented vegetables to support a healthy balance of gut bacteria.

10. Hydrate Adequately: Drink plenty of water throughout the day to stay hydrated and support digestion, especially during flare-ups with diarrhea.

11. Consider Nutritional Supplements: Talk to your healthcare provider about incorporating nutritional supplements, such as protein powders, vitamins, and minerals, to address potential deficiencies.

12. Be Mindful of Triggers: Avoid known trigger foods and ingredients that worsen symptoms, such as spicy foods, dairy, and caffeine.

13. Incorporate Snacks: Keep nutrient-dense snacks on hand, such as nut butter and banana, yogurt, rice cakes, or homemade smoothies, to help manage hunger between meals.

14. Gradually Reintroduce Foods: If following a restricted diet during flare-ups, gradually reintroduce foods as symptoms improve to identify triggers and expand dietary options.

15. **Seek Support:** Join support groups or online communities to connect with others managing ulcerative colitis and

share meal planning and preparation tips, recipes, and experiences.

16. Consult with a Dietitian: Work with a registered dietitian who specializes in gastrointestinal health to develop personalized meal plans, address nutritional concerns, and optimize dietary management of ulcerative colitis.

By incorporating these meal planning and preparation tips into your routine, you can help manage symptoms, support digestive health, and improve overall well-being while living with ulcerative colitis.

Lifestyle Strategies for Managing Ulcerative Colitis

In addition to medical treatment and dietary adjustments, adopting lifestyle strategies can contribute to the management and overall well-being of individuals with ulcerative colitis. Here are some lifestyle tips to help manage the condition:

1. Stress Management: Practice stress-reducing techniques such as deep breathing, meditation, yoga, or mindfulness. Chronic stress can exacerbate symptoms, so finding effective stress management strategies is crucial.

2. Regular Exercise: Engage in regular physical activity, as exercise has been shown to have positive effects on mood, stress reduction, and overall well-being. Consult with healthcare professionals to determine the most suitable exercise routine based on individual health status.

3. Adequate Sleep: Prioritize getting enough quality sleep each night. Establishing a consistent sleep routine and creating a comfortable sleep environment can contribute to overall health and symptom management.

4. Stay Hydrated: Drink plenty of water to stay well-hydrated, especially during flare-ups with diarrhea. Avoid sugary or caffeinated beverages, as they can contribute to dehydration.

5. Smoking Cessation: If you smoke, consider quitting. Smoking has been associated with a more severe course of ulcerative colitis and an increased risk of complications.

6. Regular Medical Check-ups: Schedule regular check-ups with healthcare providers to monitor the condition, discuss symptoms, and adjust treatment plans as needed. Early detection of changes in disease activity is essential for effective management.

7. Mindful Eating: Pay attention to eating habits and be mindful of how different foods affect symptoms. Eating slowly, chewing food thoroughly, and being conscious of portion sizes can contribute to digestive comfort.

8. Supportive Relationships: Build a support network by connecting with friends, family, or support groups. Sharing experiences with others who have ulcerative colitis can provide emotional support and valuable insights.

9. Avoid NSAIDs: Avoid nonsteroidal anti-inflammatory drugs (NSAIDs) unless prescribed by a healthcare professional. NSAIDs can exacerbate symptoms and contribute to inflammation in the digestive tract.

10. Educate Yourself: Stay informed about ulcerative colitis, treatment options, and self-management strategies. Understanding the condition empowers individuals to actively participate in their healthcare.

11. Travel Planning: Plan ahead when traveling to ensure access to necessary medications, dietary accommodations, and healthcare resources. Carry a travel kit with essentials.

12. Work-Life Balance: Strive for a healthy work-life balance. Communicate with employers about any necessary accommodations during flare-ups and seek support from coworkers.

13. Regular Bowel Habits: Establish regular bowel habits by eating meals at consistent times each day. This can help regulate bowel movements and minimize disruption to daily activities.

14. Monitor Mental Health: Be attentive to mental health, and seek support from mental health professionals if needed. Living with a chronic condition can impact emotional well-being, and addressing mental health is an important aspect of overall care.

15. **Maintain a Symptom Diary:** Keep a symptom diary to track triggers, symptom patterns, and the effectiveness of different management strategies. This information can be valuable when working with healthcare providers to optimize care.

Individuals with ulcerative colitis may find that a combination of these lifestyle strategies, along with medical and dietary management, contributes to better overall health and an improved quality of life. It's important to work collaboratively with healthcare professionals to tailor these strategies to individual needs and circumstances.

CHAPTER SIX
Managing Flare-Ups with Diet

Managing flare-ups of ulcerative colitis with diet involves making temporary adjustments to your eating habits to help reduce symptoms and support healing. Here are some dietary strategies to consider during flare-ups:

1. Low-Residue Diet: Follow a low-residue diet, which limits high-fiber foods that can irritate the digestive tract. Focus on easily digestible foods such as refined grains, well-cooked vegetables, and lean proteins.

2. Avoid Trigger Foods: Identify and avoid trigger foods that worsen symptoms. Common triggers include spicy foods, dairy products, caffeine, and high-fat foods.

3. Stay Hydrated: Drink plenty of fluids, such as water, herbal teas, and clear broths, to prevent dehydration, especially if experiencing diarrhea.

4. Small, Frequent Meals: Eat smaller, more frequent meals throughout the day to ease the workload on the digestive system and minimize discomfort.

5. Limit Dairy: If lactose intolerant or sensitive to dairy, avoid dairy products during flare-ups or choose lactose-free alternatives.

6. Cooked and Peeled Fruits/Vegetables: Opt for cooked and peeled fruits and vegetables to make them easier to digest. Avoid raw produce and tough skins.

7. Lean Proteins: Choose lean protein sources such as poultry, fish, eggs, and tofu to minimize digestive strain.

8. Avoid Spicy Foods: Steer clear of spicy foods and seasonings, as they can irritate the digestive tract and worsen symptoms.

9. Limit High-Fat Foods: Avoid high-fat foods, fried foods, and rich sauces, as they may be harder to digest and exacerbate symptoms.

10. Nutritional Supplements: Consider taking nutritional supplements, such as liquid meal replacements or protein powders, to ensure adequate nutrition if appetite is reduced.

11. Limit Alcohol and Caffeine: Reduce or eliminate alcohol and caffeine, as they can stimulate the digestive system and worsen symptoms.

12. Manage Stress: Practice stress-reduction techniques such as deep breathing, meditation, or gentle yoga to help manage stress, which can trigger or exacerbate flare-ups.

13. Avoid Raw Nuts and Seeds: Skip raw nuts and seeds during flare-ups, as they can be difficult to digest and may aggravate symptoms.

14. Cook Foods Thoroughly: Ensure that all foods are cooked thoroughly to make them easier to digest and reduce the risk of bacterial contamination.

15. Consult with Healthcare Professionals: Work closely with your healthcare team, including gastroenterologists and dietitians, to develop a personalized plan for managing flare-ups with diet.

16. Gradual Reintroduction of Foods: Once symptoms improve, gradually reintroduce foods one at a time to identify triggers and determine tolerances.

17. Monitor Symptoms: Keep track of symptoms and dietary intake in a food diary to identify patterns and make informed decisions about which foods to include or avoid.

18. Stay Informed: Stay informed about ulcerative colitis and dietary management strategies by attending educational sessions, reading reputable sources, and seeking guidance from healthcare professionals.

19. Hygiene Practices: Practice good hygiene, including washing hands thoroughly before and after handling food, to reduce the risk of bacterial contamination and infection.

20. Stay Positive: Maintain a positive attitude and stay hopeful, knowing that flare-ups are temporary and can be managed with the right approach and support.

Managing flare-ups with diet requires patience, experimentation, and a willingness to make temporary adjustments to support healing and symptom relief. By working closely with healthcare professionals and adopting a proactive approach to dietary management, individuals with ulcerative colitis can better navigate flare-ups and optimize their overall well-being.

Conclusion

In conclusion, managing ulcerative colitis involves a multifaceted approach that encompasses medical treatment, dietary modifications, and lifestyle strategies. This chronic inflammatory bowel disease requires ongoing attention and collaboration between individuals, healthcare professionals, and support networks. Key considerations include:

• **Medical Management:** Work closely with healthcare providers, including gastroenterologists, to develop an effective treatment plan. Medications and therapies may be prescribed to control inflammation and manage symptoms.

- **Dietary Modifications:** Adopting a well-planned diet tailored to individual needs is crucial in managing ulcerative colitis. Emphasize low-residue, easily digestible foods during flare-ups and gradually reintroduce a variety of nutrient-dense foods during periods of remission.

- **Lifestyle Strategies:** Incorporate stress management techniques, regular exercise, and sufficient sleep into your routine to support overall well-being. A balanced lifestyle can positively impact both physical and mental health.

- **Monitoring and Awareness:** Keep track of symptoms, triggers, and dietary intake through a symptom diary. Regular monitoring allows for better understanding of the condition and aids in making informed decisions about lifestyle, diet, and treatment adjustments.

• **Hydration and Nutritional Support:** Stay well-hydrated and consider nutritional supplements if necessary, especially during flare-ups when appetite may be reduced. Adequate nutrition is vital for supporting overall health and recovery.

• **Individualized Approach:** Recognize that each person's experience with ulcerative colitis is unique. A personalized approach to treatment, diet, and lifestyle management is essential for optimizing outcomes and quality of life.

- **Consultation with Healthcare Professionals:** Regularly consult with healthcare professionals, including gastroenterologists, dietitians, and mental health professionals. Open communication ensures that the treatment plan is tailored to your specific needs and any adjustments can be made as necessary.

- **Positive Outlook:** Maintain a positive attitude and seek support from friends, family, and support groups. Coping with a chronic condition can be challenging, but a positive mindset contributes to resilience and better overall well-being.

Ulcerative colitis management is an ongoing journey that requires adaptability and collaboration between individuals and their healthcare teams. By actively participating in the management of the condition and making informed decisions, individuals with ulcerative colitis can lead fulfilling lives, minimizing the impact of symptoms and optimizing their overall health.

THE END